45 Muscle Cramp Reduction Meal Recipes:

Eliminate Muscle Cramps for Good Using Smart Nutrition and Precise Vitamin Intake

By

Joe Correa CSN

COPYRIGHT

ACKNOWLEDGEMENTS

This book is dedicated to my friends and family that have had mild or serious illnesses so that you may find a solution and make the necessary changes in your life.

45 Muscle Cramp Reduction Meal Recipes:

Eliminate Muscle Cramps for Good Using Smart Nutrition and Precise Vitamin Intake

By

Joe Correa CSN

CONTENTS

ABOUT THE AUTHOR

After years of Research, I honestly believe in the positive effects that proper nutrition can have over the body and mind. My knowledge and experience has helped me live healthier throughout the years and which I have shared with family and friends. The more you know about eating and drinking healthier, the sooner you will want to change your life and eating habits.

Nutrition is a key part in the process of being healthy and living longer so get started today. The first step is the most important and the most significant.

INTRODUCTION

45 Muscle Cramp Reduction Meal Recipes: Eliminate Muscle Cramps for Good Using Smart Nutrition and Precise Vitamin Intake

By Joe Correa CSN

Muscle cramps are an uncomfortable experience that we all have gone through at least once in our lifetime. That awful feeling usually comes out of nowhere without any warning signs. It's basically the contraction of one or more muscles caused by the repetitive firing of neurons and nerves. But if you're experiencing muscle cramps more than usual, than it's time to learn how to solve this problem and how to treat it.

Dehydration plays an important role in this painful condition. Athletes often have this problem. Certain health problems like vomiting or diarrhea create and imbalance of electrolytes, and as a result, we have those nasty cramps. **One of the best ways to control muscle cramps is by changing your eating habits.**

As always, many health problems can be solved by putting the right kinds of foods in your kitchen. Poor nutrition and a lack of certain nutrients like calcium, potassium, magnesium, and sodium are some of the main causes of muscle cramps. Making some changes in the way you eat is the first step towards fixing this problem once and for all.

This book is a collection of fantastic recipes. It's based on super nutrient boosters that will prevent and cure muscle cramps quickly and effectively. It is an ideal collection for those who are looking for a solution through a delicious and non-restrictive diet.

These recipes are extremely rich in many different minerals that are crucial to maintain your body-fluid balance and to help normalize muscle contractions. For example, "Avocado Papaya Smoothie", "Spinach Salad", or "Vegetable Strudel" are some amazingly delicious recipes that provide you with the right sources of potassium and the best possible option to prevent this muscle cramps. **Potassium deficiency is one of the most common reasons for muscle cramps.** Even my delicious "Tuna Steak" recipe has a delightful avocado relish to help you absorb you this important mineral.

Vegetables like potatoes and pumpkin are also proven to help with muscle cramps. This is exactly why I wanted to share with you my amazing "Potato Pie", "Pumpkin Muffins", and "Potato Soup" recipes. These recipes will show you how to help yourself and enjoy a delicious meal at the same time!

Sodium is an essential mineral that is in charge of balancing blood pressure and also the mainteinance of normal body-fluid, nerve impulses, and muscle contractions. The main source of sodium in our diet is sodium chloride, known as a kitchen salt. Salted foods are everywhere around us, but large amounts of salt from processed food can be harmful to your health. **Ideally, you want to eat foods that contain natural sodium sources like cheese, celery, carrots, fish, and olives.**

In this book, you will find lots of creamy cheese recipes that are abundant in calcium. This important mineral is proven to help prevent muscle cramps.

Muscle cramps are not a serious condition. They can be treated easily through proper diet. Let this book serve as a guide to a healthier and tastier lifestyle. Try these recipes and forget about muscle cramps once and for all!

45 MUSCLE CRAMP REDUCTION MEAL RECIPES: ELIMINATE MUSCLE CRAMPS FOR GOOD USING SMART NUTRITION AND PRECISE VITAMIN INTAKE

1.   Potato Pie

Ingredients:

3 medium-sized potatoes, peeled and shredded

6 oz of cheddar cheese, crumbled

1 cup of skim milk

1 medium-sized onion, diced

½ tsp of salt

¼ tsp of black pepper, ground

2 large eggs

1 tbsp of vegetable oil

Preparation:

Preheat the oven to 350°F.

Combine potatoes and cheese in a large bowl. Stir well and spread over a previously greased baking sheet. Press equally to make a fine pie crust.

Combine eggs and onion and stir well. Pour over the crust and bake for 45 minutes. Remove from the pan if a knife inserted in the center comes out clean. Set aside to cool for 5 minutes.

Top with some extra shredded cheese for extra calcium and serve!

Nutrition information per serving: Kcal: 209, Protein: 17.6g, Carbs: 26.8g, Fats: 10.3g

2.   Berry Mix Smoothie

Ingredients:

¼ cup of strawberries, chopped

¼ cup of frozen raspberries

¼ cup of frozen blueberries

1 tbsp of honey

1 tsp of lemon juice

Preparation:

Combine all ingredients in a blender and blend until smooth. Transfer to a serving glass.

Serve with ice cubes or refrigerate for an hour before serving.

Nutrition information per serving: Kcal: 163, Protein: 2.1g, Carbs: 42.7g, Fats: 0.2g

3.   Perch with Pasta

Ingredients:

1 lb of perch, boneless and cubed (can be replaced with other white fish)

8 oz of pasta

2 cups of tomato sauce

2 tbsp of olive oil

2 tbsp of lemon juice

1 tsp of balsamic vinegar

1 garlic clove, crushed

1 tsp of vegetable mix seasoning

2 tbsp of fresh parsley, finely chopped

Preparation:

Use the package instructions to prepare the pasta. Drain well and set aside.

Heat up the oil in a large skillet over a medium-high temperature. Add garlic and saute for 2 minutes, or until translucent. Add chopped fish and season with pepper, vegetable seasoning mix, and lemon juice. Cook until fish is nearly done. Pour in the tomato sauce and reduce temperature to low. Simmer for 10-15 minutes. Remove from the heat.

Add pasta to the skillet. Give it a good stir to coat pasta with sauce and juices. Drizzle with vinegar and fresh parsley. Serve.

Nutrition information per serving: Kcal: 277, Protein: 23.9g, Carbs: 22.5g, Fats: 10.2g

4.   Spinach Salad

Ingredients:

8 oz of spinach, roughly chopped

8 oz of strawberries, halved

1 medium-sized red onion, sliced

1 medium-sized cucumber, sliced

2 tbsp of almonds, chopped

2 tbsp of lemon juice

1 tbsp of apple cider vinegar

1 tbsp of olive oil

1 tbsp of honey

¼ tsp of salt

Preparation:

Combine lemon juce, vinegar, oil, honey, and salt in a mixing bowl. Stir well and set aside to allow flavors to mingle.

Combine spinach, strawberries, onion, cucumber, and almonds in a large salad bowl. Drizzle with dressing and toss well before serving.

Nutrition information per serving: Kcal: 142, Protein: 4.3g, Carbs: 21.7g, Fats: 7.2g

5.   Chocolate Cranberry Smoothie

Ingredients:

¼ cup of chocolate chips

½ cup of skim milk

6 oz of vanilla yogurt

1 cup of fresh cranberries

Preparation:

Combine all ingredients in a food processor. Blend for one minute or until smooth. Transfer to a serving glasses and add some ice. You can use frozen berries instead of ice.

Top with shredded dark chocolate.

Nutrition information per serving: Kcal: 461, Protein: 13.1g, Carbs: 71.7g, Fats: 10.3g

6.   Banana Peppers

Ingredients:

10 banana sweet peppers

1 lb of ground lean beaf

¼ cup of all-purpose flour

½ cup of Swiss cheese, shredded

1 medium-sized onion, chopped

1 tsp of vegetable oil

1 large egg

¼ tsp of black pepper, ground

Preparation:

Preheat the oven to 350°F.

Heat the oil in a large frying pan over a medium-high temperature. Add the onion, and stir-fry until golden brown. Add the meat and cook until nicely brown. Stir in the cheese and cook for 2 minutes more. Remove from the heat and set aside to cool for a while.

Clean the peppers, removing top and bottom parts. Stuff the peppers with meat mixture.

Beat the egg and combine with pepper in a mixing bowl. Dip the stuffed peppers in egg mixture. Coat with flour, dip in egg, and coat again.

Spray the baking sheet with some vegetable oil and place the peppers. Bake for about 20 minutes.

Top with sour cream, but this is, however optional.

Nutrition information per serving: Kcal: 385, Protein: 29.3g, Carbs: 18.3g, Fats: 15.4g

7.   Potato Soup

Ingredients:

3 medium-sized potatoes, peeled and mashed

3 tbsp of Parmesan cheese, shredded

½ cup of celery, finely chopped

1 tsp of fresh parsley, finely chopped

1 medium-sized onion, sliced

1 medium-sized carrot, sliced

12 oz of chicken broth

4 oz of milk, non-fat

1 tbsp of all-purpose flour

1 tsp of salt

Preparation:

Combine all ingredients in a slow cooker, except cheese and milk. Cover with a lid and cook for 7 hours on a medium heat.

Combine flour and milk in a mixing bowl and whisk well. Pour it into the cooker and sprinkle with shredded cheese. Cook for another 20 minutes without lid.

Serve warm.

Nutrition information per serving: Kcal: 324, Protein: 5.3g, Carbs: 28.3g, Fats: 7.3g

8.   Salmon Croquettes

Ingredients:

12 oz of wild salmon, skinless and boneless

3 tbsp of breadcrumps

2 grain bread slices

5 tbsp of mayonnaise

1 medium-sized onion, chopped

1 small bell pepper, chopped

½ tsp of salt

¼ tsp of black pepper, ground

Preparation:

Preheat the oven to 400°F.

Combine all ingredients except breadcrumps in a large bowl. Stir well to combine. Using hands, shape the croquettes and coat well with breadcrumbs.

Line some baking paper over a baking sheet and place the croquettes. Bake for about 20 minutes and remove from the oven.

Serve warm.

Nutrition information per serving: Kcal: 137, Protein: 15.3g, Carbs: 10.4g, Fats: 11.3g

9.   Pumpkin muffins

Ingredients:

2 cups of pumpkin pie mix

1 cup of flour, whole wheat

¼ cup of milk, low-fat

2 tbsp of oat meal

2 large eggs

½ cup of applesauce

¼ cup of raisins

½ cup of walnuts, finely chopped

1 tsp of baking powder

1 tsp of vanilla extract

1 tbsp of butter

1 tsp of baking soda

Preparation:

Preheat the oven to 350°F.

Mix flour, baking powder, oats and soda in a large mixing bowl. Add pumpkin mix and stir all well together to combine. Set aside.

Now, combine raisins, walnuts, milk, butter, applesauce, and vanilla extract in a separate bowl. Stir well to combine. Now, combine both mixtures and give it a good stir.

Fill up lightly greased muffin molds with batter and put it in the oven.

Bake for 25 minutes and remove from the oven. Let it cool for about 15 minutes and serve.

Top with chocolate or cinnamon sprinkle.

Nutrition information per serving: Kcal: 172, Protein: 2.4g, Carbs: 38.8g, Fats: 8.9g

10.   Smoked Gouda Omelet

Ingredients:

3 tbsp of smoked gouda cheese, shredded

1 free-range egg

4 egg whites

1 medium-sized onion, sliced

1 tsp of yellow mustard

2 tbsp of skim milk

2 tsp of vegetable oil

Preparation:

Preheat 1 teaspoon of oil in a large frying pan over a medium-high temperature. add the onion and stir-fry until translucent. You can add a tablespoon of water to get more juice. Transfer the onion to a mixing bowl and stir in the mustard. Set aside.

Preheat remaining oil over a medium temperature. Meanwhile, combine milk, egg, and whites. Whisk well and pour the mixture into the skillet. Cook until eggs are nearly done. Spread the onion and gouda cheese over one half of the omelet. Flip over another half and cook for 2minutes more. Remove from the heat and cut into portions. Serve.

Nutrition information per serving: Kcal: 201, Protein: 13.5g, Carbs: 18.7g, Fats: 8.8g

11. Leek and Carrot Soup

Ingredients:

1 cup of leeks, chopped

1 medium-sized potato, peeled and sliced

2 medium-sized carrots, sliced

1 cup of chicken broth

2 cups of skim milk

1 cup of corn, frozen

2 tbsp of fresh parsley, finely chopped

½ tsp of salt

¼ tsp of black pepper, ground

Preparation:

Mix together leeks, potato, carrots in a large pot. Pour in vegetable broth and sprinkle with salt and pepper. Cover with a lid and cook for about 10-15 minutes, or until fork-tender.

Now, add corn and milk and simmer for 5 minutes. Remove from the heat transfer to a serving bowls.

Sprinkle with parsley and serve.

Nutrition information per serving: Kcal: 241, Protein: 13.2g, Carbs: 43.6g, Fats: 8.3g

12.   Catfish with Pecans

Ingredients:

1 lb of catfish fillets

1 cup of pecans, ground

½ cup of skim milk

1 tbsp of olive oil

6 tbsp of Dijon mustard

1 tbsp of lemon juice

3 small potatoes, peeled and cubed

Preparation:

Preheat the oven to 400°F.

Put potatoes in a pot of boiling water. Sprinkle with vegetable seasoning mix and cook until fork-tender. Drain and set aside to cool for a while.

Combine mustard and milk in a mixing bowl. Dipp fish fillets in the mixture then coat with pecans. Place the fillets on a greased baking sheet and put it in the oven. Bake for 10-12 minutes. remove from the oven and serve with potatoes.

Drizzle potatoes with lemon juice and serve.

Nutrition information per serving: Kcal: 438, Protein: 24.4g, Carbs: 25.7g, Fats: 38.3g

13.   Avocado Papaya Smoothie

Ingredients:

1 papaya, chopped

½ avocado, chopped

1 cup of plain yogurt, fat-free

1 tsp of coconut extract

1 tsp of flaxseeds, ground

Preparation:

Combine all inredients in a food processor except flaxseeds. Blend for 1 minute or until smooth. Transfer to a serving glasses and top with flaxseeds. Refigerate 30 minutes before serving.

Nutrition information per serving: Kcal: 380, Protein: 15.1g, Carbs: 68.2g, Fats: 10.7g

14. Tuna Steaks

Ingredients:

4 tuna steaks, about 6 oz each

½ tsp of lime zest, finely grated

1 garlic clove, crushed

2 tsp olive oil

1 tsp of cumin, ground

1 tsp of coriander, ground

¼ tsp of black pepper, ground

1 tbsp lime juice

For avocado relish:

1 tbsp of fresh coriander, chopped

1 small avocado, pitted, peeled and chopped

1 small red onion, finely chopped

Preparation:

Trim the skin from the tuna steaks, then rinse and pat dry on absorbent kitchen paper.

In a small bowl, mix together the lime zest, garlic, olive oil, cumin, ground coriander and pepper to make a paste.

Spread the paste thinly on both sides of the tuna. Cook the tuna steaks for 5 minutes, turning once, on a foil-covered barbecue rack over hot coals, or in an oiled, ridged grill pan over high heat, in batches if necessary. Cook for another 4-5 minutes, drain on kitchen paper and transfer to a serving plate.

Sprinkle the lime juice and sprigs of fresh coriander over the cooked fish. Serve the tuna steaks with avocado relish and wedges of lime and tomato.

Avocado Relish:

To make avocado relish, peel and chop small, ripe avocado. Mix in 1 tablespoon of lime juice, 1 tablespoon of freshly chopped coriander, 1 small, finely chopped red onion and some fresh mango or tomato. Season to taste.

Nutrition information per serving: Kcal: 239, Protein: 42.3g, Carbs: 0.5g, Fats: 8.4g

15.   Vegetarian Chili Beans

Ingredients:

2 small fresh red chillies, finely chopped

1 medium-sized green bell pepper, diced

14 oz can red kidney beans, rinsed

14 oz can tomatoes, diced

4 oz of tomato pasta sauce

1 tbsp of vegetable oil

2 garlic cloves, crushed

Preparation:

Heat the oil in a heavy-based pan and cook the garlic, chilli and onion for 3 minutes, or until the onion is golden.

Add the remaining ingredients, bring to a boil, then reduce the heat to simmer for 15 minutes, or until thickened.

Nutrition information per serving: Kcal: 190, Protein: 9.4g, Carbs: 34.5g, Fats: 1.6g

16.   Vegetable Strudel

Ingredients:

1 large eggplant

1 medium-sized red bell pepper, chopped

3 zucchini, sliced lengthwise

2 tbsps olive oil

6 sheets filo pastry

1¾ oz baby English spinach leaves

2 oz of feta cheese, sliced

Preparation:

Slice the eggplant lengthwise. Sprinkle with salt and leave for 20 minutes (to draw out the bitterness). Rinse well and pat dry.

Cut the pepper into large flat pieces and place, skin side up, under a hot grill until the skin blackens and blisters. Put in a plastic bag, then peel the skin away. Brush the eggplant and zucchini slices with some of the olive oil and grill for 5-10 minutes, or until golden brown. Set aside to cool. Preheat the oven to moderately hot, about 375°F.

Brush one sheet of filo pastry at a time with olive oil, then lay them on top of each other. Place half the eggplant slices lengthwise down the center of the filo and top with layers of zucchini, pepper, spinach and feta cheese. Repeat the layers until the vegetable and cheese are used up. Tuck in the ends of the pastry, then roll up like a parcel. Brush lightly with oil, place on a baking tray and bake for 35 minutes, or until golden brown.

Nutrition information per serving: Kcal: 287, Protein: 16.3g, Carbs: 38.2g, Fats: 2.8g

17. Stuffed Field Mushrooms

Ingredients:

4 large field mushrooms

1 oz of butter

1 leek, sliced

3 garlic cloves, crushed

2 tsp of cumin seeds

1 tsp fresh coriander, ground

¼ tsp of chilli powder

2 medium-sized tomatoes, chopped

2 cups of mixed vegetables, frozen

½ cup of white rice, pre-cooked

1 oz of Cheddar cheese, grated

¼ cup Parmesan cheese, grated

¼ cup of cashews, chopped

Preparation:

Preheat the oven to 400°F. Wipe the mushrooms with a paper towel. Remove the stalks and chop them finely.

Melt the butter in a pan. Add the chopped mushroom stalks and leek and cook for 2-3 minutes, or until soft. Mix in the garlic, cumin seeds, ground coriander and chilli powder and cook for 1 minute, or until the mixture is fragrant.

Stir in the tomato and frozen vegetables. Bring to a boil, reduce the heat and simmer for 5 minutes. Stir in the rice and season well.

Spoon the mixture into the mushroom caps, sprinkle with the Cheddar and Parmesan and bake for 15 minutes, or until the cheese has melted. Scatter with the cashews and serve.

Nutrition information per serving: Kcal: 180, Protein: 3.4g, Carbs: 6.6g, Fats: 3.7g

18.   Chickpea Burgers

Ingredients:

14 oz chickpeas, soaked

1 cup of red lentils

1 tbsp of vegetable oil

2 onions, sliced

1 tsp cumin, ground

1 tsp of garam masala

1 large egg

¼ cup of fresh parsley, chopped

2 tbsp fresh coriander, ground

6 oz of stale breadcrumbs

Plain flour, for dusting

Preparation:

Add the lentils to a large pan of boiling water and simmer for 8 minutes, or until tender. Drain well. Heat the oil in a pan and cook the onion for 3 minutes, or until soft. Add the ground spices and stir until fragrant. Cool the mixture slightly.

Place the chickpeas, egg, onion mixture and half the lentils in a food processor. Process for 20 seconds, or until smooth. Transfer to a bowl. Stir in the remaining lentils, parsley, coriander and breadcrumbs. Mix well. Divide into 10 portions.

Shape the portions into round patties. (If the mixture is too soft, chill for 15 minutes, or until firm.) Toss the patties in flour, shaking off the excess. Place on a lightly greased hot barbecue grill or hotplate. Cook for 3-4 minutes on each side, or until browned.

Nutrition information per serving: Kcal: 127, Protein: 5.4g, Carbs: 24.6g, Fats: 1.3g

19.   Moroccan Couscous

Ingredients:

2 tbsp olive oil

2 cloves garlic, crushed

1 small red chilli, diced

1 leek, thinly sliced

2 small fennel bulbs, sliced

2 tsp ground cumin

1 tsp ground coriander

1 tsp ground turmeric

1 tspgaram masala

11 oz sweet potato, chopped

2 parsnips, sliced

1½ cups vegetable stock

2 zucchini, thickly sliced

8 oz broccoli, cut into florets

2 tomatoes, peeled and chopped

1 red pepper, chopped

14 oz can chickpeas, drained

2 tbsp chopped fresh flat-leaf parsley

2 tbsp chopped fresh lemon thyme

Couscous:

1¼ cups instant couscous

1 oz butter

1 cup hot vegetable stock

Preparation:

Heat the oil in a large pan and add the garlic, chilli, leek and fennel. Cook over medium heat for 10 minutes, or until the leek and fennel are soft and golden brown.

Add the cumin, coriander, turmeric, garam masala, sweet potato and parsnip. Cook for 5 minutes, stirring to coat the vegetables with spices.

Add the vegetable stock and simmer, covered, for 15 minutes. Stir in the zucchini, broccoli, tomato, pepper and chickpeas. Simmer, uncovered, for 30 minutes, or until the vegetables are tender. Stir in the herbs.

Put the couscous and butter in a bowl. Pour in the stock and leave to absorb for 5 minutes. Fluff gently with a fork to separate the grains. Make the couscous into a 'nest' on each plate and serve the spicy vegetables in the middle.

Nutrition information per serving: Kcal: 219, Protein: 6.5g, Carbs: 40g, Fats: 3g

20.   Nut Roast

Ingredients:

2 tbsp olive oil

1 large onion, diced

2 cloves garlic, crushed

10 oz field mushrooms, finely chopped

6½ oz raw cashews

6½ ozbrazil nuts

1 cup grated Cheddar

¼ cup freshly grated Parmesan

1 egg, lightly beaten

2 tbsp chopped fresh chives

1 cup fresh wholemeal breadcrumbs

Tomato Sauce:

1 floz olive oil

1 onion, finely chopped

1 clove garlic, crushed

13 fire roasted tomatoes, chopped

1 tbsp tomato paste

1 tsp caster sugar

Preparation:

Grease a 5½ x 8½ inches loaf tin and line the base with baking paper. Heat the oil in a frying pan and add the onion, garlic and mushrooms. Fry until soft, then allow to cool.

Process the nuts in a food processor until finely chopped, but do not overprocess. Preheat the oven to moderate 350 degrees.

Mix together the nuts, mushroom mixture, cheese, egg, chives and breadcrumbs. Press firmly into the loaf tin and bake for 15 minutes, or until firm. Leave in the tin for 5 minutes, then turn out.

To make the sauce, heat the oil in a pan and add the onion and garlic. Fry for 5 minutes, or until soft but not brown. Add the chopped tomatoes, tomato paste, sugar and 1/3 cup of water. Simmer for 3-5 minutes, or until the sauce has slightly thickened. Season to taste with salt and pepper. Serve the tomato sauce with the sliced nut roast.

Nutrition information per serving: Kcal: 297, Protein: 12g, Carbs: 24g, Fats: 14g

21.   Tomato Salsa Chickpeas

Ingredients:

2 cups chickpeas

1 small onion, chopped

2 cloves garlic, crushed

2 tbsp chopped fresh parsley

1 tbsp chopped fresh coriander

2 tsp ground cumin

½ tsp baking powder

Oil, for deep-frying

Hummus:

14 oz chickpeas

2-3 tbsp lemon juice

2 tbsp olive oil

2 cloves garlic, crushed

3 tbsp tahini

Tomato salsa:

2 tomatoes, peeled and finely chopped

¼ cucumber, finely chopped

½ green pepper, finely chopped

2 tbsp chopped fresh parsley

1 tsp sugar

2 tspchilli sauce

Grated rind and juice of 1 lemon

Preparation:

Soak the chickpeas in 3 cups of water for at least 4 hours. Drain and mix in a food processor for 30 seconds, or until finely ground.

Add the onion, garlic, parsley, coriander, cumin, baking powder and 1 tbsp water, and process for 10 seconds, or until the mixture forms a rough paste. Cover and set aside for 30 minutes.

To make the hummus, place the drained chickpeas, lemon juice, oil and garlic in a food processor. Season and process for 20-30 seconds, or until smooth. Add the tahini and process for a further 10 seconds.

To make the tomato salsa, mix together all the ingredients and season with plenty of freshly ground black pepper.

Shape heaped tablespoons of the falafel mixture into balls. Squeeze out the excess moisture. Heat the oil in a deep, heavy-based pan, until a cube of bread browns in 15 seconds. Lower the falafel into the oil in batches of five. Cook for 3-4 minutes each batch. When well-browned, remove with a large slotted spoon. Drain on paper towels and serve hot or cold with Lebanese bread, hummus and tomato salsa.

Nutrition information per serving: Kcal: 150, Protein: 3.9g, Carbs: 15.2g, Fats: 6g

22.   Steamed Potato Frittata

Ingredients:

1 tbsp olive oil

2 cloves garlic, crushed

1 small red onion, chopped

1 small red pepper, chopped

1 lb roasted, boiled or steamed potatoes, thickly sliced

¼ cup chopped fresh parsley

6 eggs, lightly beaten

¼ cup grated Parmesan

Preparation:

Heat the oil in a large, heavy-based, non-stick frying pan. Add the garlic, onion and pepper and stir over medium heat for 2-3 minutes. Add the potato slices and cook for 2-3 minutes more. Stir in the parsley and spread the mixture evenly in the pan.

Beat the eggs with 2 tbsp water, pour into the pan and cook over medium heat for 15 minutes, without burning the base.

Preheat the grill to high. Sprinkle the Parmesan over the frittata and grill for a few minutes to cook the egg and lightly brown. Cut into wedges to serve.

Nutrition information per serving: Kcal: 208, Protein: 11g, Carbs: 17g, Fats: 10g

23.   Cannellini Beans Sausages

Ingredients:

1 tbsp sunflower oil

1 small onion, finely chopped

1¾ oz mushrooms, finely chopped

½ red pepper, deseeded and finely chopped

14 oz cannellini beans, rinsed and drained

3½ oz fresh breadcrumbs

3½ oz Cheddar cheese, grated

1 tsp dried mixed herbs

1 egg yolk

All-purpose flour, to coat

Oil, for cooking

Preparation:

Heat the oil in a pan and cooked the prepared onion, mushrooms and red pepper until softened.

Mash the cannellini beans in a large mixing bowl. Add the chopped onion, mushroom and red pepper mixture, and the breadcrumbs, cheese, herbs and egg yolk, and mix together well.

Press the mixture together with your fingers and shape into eight sausages.

Roll each sausage in the seasoned flour. Chill for at least 30 minutes.

Barbecue the sausages on a sheet of oiled foil set over medium-hot coals for 15-20 minutes, turning and basting frequently with oil, until golden.

Split the bread rolls down the middle and insert a layer of fried onions. Place the sausages in the rolls and serve.

Nutrition information per serving: Kcal: 213, Protein: 8g, Carbs: 19g, Fats: 12g

24. Grated Pupkin Frittata

Ingredients:

3 tbsp olive oil

1 onion, finely chopped

1 small carrot, grated

1 small zucchini, grated

1 cup grated pumpkin

1/3 cup finely-diced Cheddar cheese

5 eggs, lightly beaten

Preparation:

Heat 2 tablespoons of the oil in a pan and cook the onion for 5 minutes, or until soft. Add the carrot, zucchini and pumpkin and cook over low heat, covered, for 3 minutes. Transfer to a bowl and allow to cool. Stir in the cheese and plenty of salt and pepper. Add the eggs.

Heat the remaining oil in a small non-stick frying pan. Add the frittata mixture and shake the pan to spread it evenly. Reduce to low and cook for 15-20 minutes, or until set almost all the way through. Tilt the pan and lift the edges occasionally to allow the uncooked egg to flow underneath. Brown the top under a preheated hot grill. Cut into wedges and serve immediately.

Nutrition information per serving: Kcal: 114, Protein: 10g, Carbs: 6g, Fats: 5g

25.   Colorful Kebabs

Ingredients:

1 red pepper, deseeded

1 yellow pepper, deseeded

1 green pepper, deseeded

1 small onion

8 cherry tomatoes

3½ oz wild mushrooms

Seasoned oil:

6 tbsp olive oil

1 garlic clove, crushed

½ tsp mixed dried herbs

Preparation:

Cut the red, yellow and green peppers into 1-inch pieces.

Peel the onion and cut into wedges, leaving the root end just intact to help keep the wedges together.

Thread the pepper pieces, onion wedges, tomatoes and mushrooms onto skewers, alternating the colors of the peppers.

To make the seasoned oil, mix together the olive oil, garlic and mixed herbs in a small bowl. Brush the mixture liberally over the kebabs.

Barbecue the kebabs over medium-hot coals for 10-15 minutes, brushing with the seasoned oil and turning the skewers frequently.

Transfer the vegetable kebabs onto warmed serving plates.

Nutrition information per serving: Kcal: 257, Protein: 3g, Carbs: 26g, Fats: 16g

26.   Garlic Potato Wedges

Ingredients:

3 large baking potatoes, scrubbed

4 tbsp olive oil

2 tbsp butter

2 garlic cloves, chopped

1 tbsp chopped fresh rosemary

1 tbsp chopped fresh parsley

1 tbsp chopped fresh thyme

Salt and pepper

Preparation:

Bring a large saucepan of water to a boil, add the potatoes and parboil them for 10 minutes. Drain the potatoes, refresh under cold water and then drain them again thoroughly.

Transfer the potatoes to a chopping board. When cold enough to handle, cut into thick wedges, but do not peel.

Heat the oil, butter and garlic in a small saucepan. Cook gently until the garlic begins to brown, then remove the pan from the heat.

Stir the herbs, and salt and pepper to taste, into the mixture in the saucepan.

Brush the warm garlic and herb mixture generously over the parboiled potato wedges.

Barbecue the potatoes over hot coals for 10-15 minutes, brushing liberally with any of the remaining garlic and herb mixture, or until the potato wedges are just tender.

Transfer the garlic potato wedges to a warm serving plate and serve as a starter or side dish.

Nutrition information per serving: Kcal: 336, Protein: 3.9g, Carbs: 32.4g, Fats: 26.8g

27.   Saffron Risotto

Ingredients:

Large pinch of good-quality saffron threads

16 floz boiling water

1 tsp salt

2 tbsp butter

2 tbsp olive oil

1 large onion, very finely chopped

3 tbsp pine kernels

12 oz long grain rice

2oz sultanas

6 green cardamom pods, shells lightly cracked

6 cloves

Pepper

Very finely chopped fresh coriander or flat-leaved parsley, to garnish

Preparation:

Toast the saffron threads in a dry frying pan over a medium heat, stirring, for 2 minutes, until they give off an aroma. Immediately tip out onto a plate.

Pour the boiling water into a measuring jug, stir in the saffron and salt and leave to infuse for 30 minutes.

Melt the butter and oil in a frying pan over a medium-high heat. Add the onion. Cook for about 5 minutes, stirring.

Lower the heat, stir the pine kernels into the onions and continue cooking for 2 minutes, stirring, until the nuts just begin to turn a golden color. Take care not to burn them.

Stir in the rice, coating all the grains with oil. Stir for 1 minute, then add the sultanas, cardamom pods and cloves. Pour in the saffron-flavored water and bring to a boil. Lower the heat, cover and simmer for 15 minutes without removing the lid.

Remove from the heat. Leave to stand for 5 minutes without uncovering. Remove the lid and check that the rice is tender, the liquid has been absorbed and the surface has small indentations all over.

Fluff up the rice and adjust the seasoning. Stir in the herbs and serve.

Nutrition information per serving: Kcal: 347, Protein: 5g, Carbs: 60g, Fats: 11g

28.   Ginger Charred Chicken

Ingredients:

4 chicken breasts, skinned and boned

2 tbsp curry paste

1 tbsp sunflower oil, plus extra for cooking

1 tbsp brown sugar

1 tsp ground ginger

½ tsp ground cumin

Yogurt Topping:

¼ cucumber

Salt

½ cup of low-fat natural yogurt

¼ tsp chilli powder

Preparation:

Place the chicken breasts between two sheets of baking paper or clingfilm. Pound them with the flat side of a meat mallet or rolling pin to flatten them. Mix together the curry paste, oil, brown sugar, ginger and cumin in a small bowl.

Spread the mixture over both sides of the chicken and then set aside until required.

To make the yogurt topping, peel the cucumber and scoop out the seeds with a spoon. Grate the cucumber flesh, sprinkle with salt, place in a sieve and leave to stand for 10 minutes. Rinse off the salt and squeeze out any remaining moisture by pressing the cucumber with the base of a glass or the back of a spoon. In a small bowl, mix the grated cucumber with the natural yogurt and stir in the chilli powder. Leave to chill until needed.

Transfer the chicken pieces to an oiled rack and barbecue over hot coals for 10 minutes, turning once.

Serve the chicken with yogurt topping.

Nutrition information per serving: Kcal: 228, Protein: 28g, Carbs: 12g, Fats: 8g

29.   Apples Stuffed with Nuts and Cherries

Ingredients:

4 medium cooking apples

2 tbsp chopped walnuts

2 tbsp ground almonds

2 tbsp light muscovado sugar

2 tbsp chopped cherries

2 tbsp chopped crystallized ginger

4 tbsp butter

Single cream or thick natural yogurt, to serve

Preparation:

Core the apples and, using a sharp knife, score each one around the middle to prevent the apple skins from splitting during barbecuing.

To make the filling, in a small bowl, mix together the walnuts, almonds, sugar, cherries and ginger.

Spoon the filling mixture into each apple, pushing it down into the hollowed-out core. Mound a little of the filling mixture on top of each apple.

Place each apple on a large square of double-thickness foil and generously dot with the butter. Wrap up the foil so that each apple is completely enclosed.

Barbecue the parcels containing the apples over hot coals for about 25-30 minutes, or until tender.

Transfer the apples to warm individual serving plates. Serve with lashings of whipped single cream or thick natural yogurt.

Nutrition information per serving: Kcal: 294, Protein: 3g, Carbs: 31g, Fats: 18g

30.   Creamy Banana Dessert

Ingredients:

4 bananas

2 passionfruit

4 tbsp orange juice

4 tbsp orange-flavored liqueur

Creamy topping:

5 floz double cream

3 tbsp icing sugar

2 tbsp orange-flavored liqueur

Preparation:

To make the orange-flavored cream, pour the double cream into a mixing bowl and sprinkle over the icing sugar. Whisk the mixture until it is standing in soft peaks. Carefully fold in the orange-flavored liqueur and chill in the refrigerator until needed.

Peel the bananas and place each one onto a sheet of foil.

Cut the passion fruit in half and squeeze the juice of each half over each banana. Spoon over the orange juice and liqueur. Fold the foil carefully over the top of the bananas so that they are completely enclosed.

Place the parcels on a baking tray and cook over hot coals for 10-15 minutes, or until they are just tender (test by inserting a cocktail stick or a toothpick). Transfer the foil parcels to warm, individual serving plates. Open out the foil parcels and then serve immediately with the orange-flavored cream.

Nutrition information per serving: Kcal: 380, Protein: 2g, Carbs: 43g, Fats: 19g

31.   Thick Red Lentil Soup

Ingredients:

2 tbsp butter

2 garlic cloves, crushed

1 onion, chopped

½ tsp turmeric

1 tsp garam masala

¼ tsp chilli powder

1 tsp ground cumin

2 lb of chopped tomatoes

7 oz red lentils

2 tsp lemon juice

1 pint vegetable stock

10 floz coconut milk

Salt and pepper

For serving:

Fresh chopped coriander

Lemon slices

Preparation:

Melt the butter in a large saucepan. Add the garlic and onion and saute, stirring, for 2-3 minutes. Add the turmeric, garam masala, chilli powder and cumin and cook for another 30 seconds.

Chop the tomatoes and stir into the pan with the red lentils, lemon juice, vegetable stock and coconut stock and bring to a boil.

Reduce the heat to low and simmer the soup, uncovered for about 25-30 minutes until the lentils are tender and cooked.

Season to taste with salt and pepper and ladle the soup into warm serving bowls. Garnish with chopped coriander and lemon slices and serve immediately with warm naan bread.

Nutrition information per serving: Kcal: 284, Protein: 16g, Carbs: 38g, Fats: 9g

32.   Chicken Soup

Ingredients:

12oz minced chicken

1 tbsp tomato sauce

1 tsp grated fresh root ginger

1 garlic clove, finely chopped

2 tsp sherry

2 spring onions, chopped

1 tsp sesame oil

1 egg white

½ tsp corn flour

½ tsp sugar

35 wonton skins

2½ pints chicken stock

1 spring onion, shredded

1 small carrot, thinly sliced

Preparation:

Put the chicken, ginger, garlic, sherry, spring onions, sesame oil, egg white, cornflour and sugar in a bowl and mix well. Place a small spoonful of the filling in the center of each wonton skin. Dampen the edges. Gather up each one to form a pouch to enclose the filling.

Cook the wontons in boiling water for 1 minute or until they float to the surface. Remove with a slotted spoon.

Pour the chicken stock into a saucepan and bring to a boil. Add the spring onion, carrot and wontons to the soup. Simmer gently for 2 minutes, then serve.

Nutrition information per serving: Kcal: 101, Protein: 14g, Carbs: 3g, Fats: 4g

33.   Tomato Kebabs

Ingredients:

1 lb rump or sirloin steak

16 cherry tomatoes

16 large green olives, stoned

Salt and freshly ground black pepper

Focaccia bread, to serve

4 tbsp olive oil

1 tbsp sherry vinegar

1 garlic clove, crushed

1 tbsp olive oil

1 tbsp sherry vinegar

1 garlic clove, crushed

6 plum tomatoes, skinned, deseeded anc chopped

2 green olives, stoned and sliced

1 tbsp chopped fresh parsley

1 tbsp lemon juice

Preparation:

Trim any fat from the meat and cut into about 24 even-sized pieces.Thread the meat into 8 skewers, alternating it with cherry tomatoes and the stoned whole olives.

To make the baste, in a bowl combine the oil, vinegar, garlic, and salt and pepper to taste.

To make the fresh tomato relish, heat the oil in a small saucepan and cook the onion and garlic for 3-4 minutes until softened. Add the tomatoes and sliced olives and cook for 2-3 minutes until the tomatoes are softened slightly. Stir in the parsley and lemon juice, and season with salt and pepper to taste. Set aside and keep warm or leave to chill.

Barbecue the skewers on an oiled rack over hot coals for 5-10 minutes, basting and turning frequently. Serve with the tomato relish and slices of focaccia.

Nutrition information per serving: Kcal: 166, Protein: 12g, Carbs: 1g, Fats: 12g

34.   Pork with Rice

Ingredients:

14oz lean pork fillet

3 tbsp orange marmalade

Grated zest and juice of 1 orange

1 tbsp white wine vinegar

1 tsp of Tabasco sauce

Salt and pepper

1 tbsp olive oil

1 small onion, chopped

1 small, green pepper, deseeded and thinly sliced

1 tbspcornflour

5 floz orange juice

Serving:

Cooked rice

Mixed salad leaves

Preparation:

Place a large piece of double thickness foil in a shallow dish. Put the pork fillet in the center of the foil and season to taste. Heat the marmalade, orange zest and juice, vinegar and Tabasco sauce in a small pan, stirring, until the marmalade melts and the ingredients combine. Pour the mixture over the pork and wrap the meat in the foil. Seal the parcel well so that the juices cannot run out. Place over hot coals and barbecue for 25 minutes, turning the parcel occasionally.

For the sauce, heat the oil in a pan and cook the onion for 2-3 minutes. Add the pepper and cook for 3-4 minutes. Remove the pork from the foil and place on the racke. Pour the juices into the pan with the sauce. Continue barbecuing the pork for another 10-20 minutes, turning, until cooked through and golden.

In a bowl, mix the cornflour into a paste with a little orange juice. Add to the sauce with the remaining cooking juices. Cook, stirring, until it thickens. Slice the pork, spoon over the sauce and serve with rice and salad leaves.

Nutrition information per serving: Kcal: 230, Protein: 19g, Carbs: 16g, Fats: 9g

35.   French Croissant

Ingredients:

2 pounds of all-purpose flour

1 small pack of dry yeast

2 tsp salt

5 tbsp oil

1 whole egg

1 ½ cup of milk

1 cup of water

1 cup butter

1 whole egg

1 egg yolk

1 cup of organic cocoa cream

Preparation:

In a small bowl combine the yeast with 1/2 cup of warm milk, 1 tsp of sugar, and 1 tsp of all-purpose flour. Allow it to stand for about 30 minutes. Combine the yeast with other ingredients and make a smooth dough. Shape 16 little bowls and roll out the dough.

Place 1 tbsp of cocoa cream at the center of each croissant and roll in.

Preheat the oven to 400 degrees and bake the croissants for about 15 minutes.

Meanwhile, combine 1 egg and 1 egg yolk in a bowl. Spread this mixture, with a kitchen brush, over each croissant before removing them from the oven.

Nutrition information per serving: Kcal: 491, Protein: 10g, Carbs: 59g, Fats: 23.5g

36.   Seafood Risotto with Turmeric

Ingredients:

1 cup of rice

1 cup of fresh seafood mix

½ cup of peas, cooked

1 small tomato

½ bell pepper, finely chopped

1 tbsp of ground turmeric

Salt to taste

Preparation:

Briefly boil the seafood mix, for about 3-4 minutes. Drain and set aside.

Add one cup of rice and 3 cups of water in a deep pot. Bring it to a boil and cook for about 10 minutes, or until half of the water has evaporated.

Meanwhile, peel and finely chop the tomato and bell pepper. Mix with peas in a bowl and season with salt.

Combine this mixture with rice, add seafood mix, one tablespoon of ground turmeric and cook until all the water has evaporated. You can serve with some grated Parmesan cheese.

Nutrition information per serving: Kcal: 198, Protein: 4.8g, Carbs: 42.7g, Fats: 0.6g

37. Lentil and Chickpea Salad with Fresh Lemon Juice

Ingredients:

½ cup of cooked lentils

½ cup of cooked chickpeas

½ red onion, finely chopped

1 cup of lettuce, finely chopped

3 tbsp of fresh lemon juice

2 tbsp of olive oil

Preparation:

First you will have to cook the lentils. For ½ cup of dry lentils, you will need 1 ½ cup of water, because the lentils will double in size. Bring it to a boil, reduce the heat and cook for about 15-20 minutes, or until the lentils have softened. Remove from the heat and drain. Allow it to cool for a while.

Place all the ingredients in a bowl and mix well. Before serving, add three tablespoons of fresh lemon juice and two tablespoons of olive oil. Toss well to coat.

Nutrition information per serving: Kcal: 246, Protein: 11.3g, Carbs: 31.5g, Fats: 8.9g

38.   Quick Homemade Polenta

Ingredients:

17oz corn flour

5 cups of water

5 tbsp of olive oil

A pinch of salt

Preparation:

Bring five cups of water to a boiling point. Add salt, olive oil, and reduce the heat to medium. Slowly whisk in the corn flour. Cook until the mixture thickens, stirring often. Remove from the heat and serve.

Nutrition information per serving: Kcal: 334, Protein: 4.8g, Carbs: 52.9g, Fats: 12.7g

39.   Lean Potato Salad with Olive Oil

Ingredients:

2 medium-sized potatoes, boiled

5 spring onions, finely chopped

1 small red onion, peeled and sliced

Olive oil to taste

Salt to taste

Pepper to taste

Preparation:

First you will have to boil the potatoes. Peel and thoroughly rinse the potatoes. Slice and transfer to a deep pot. Add just enough water to cover. Bring it to a boil and cook for about 15 minutes, or until the potatoes have softened. Remove from the heat and drain. Allow it to cool for a while.

Meanwhile, prepare the onions. Trim the roots away and strip off any extra outer leaves. Finely chop and combine with potatoes.

Peel and slice the onion. Add to the salad mixture. Season with olive oil, salt and pepper to taste. You can add a few drops of fresh lemon juice, but this is optional.

Serve cold.

Nutrition information per serving: Kcal: 259, Protein: 3.1g, Carbs: 26.3g, Fats: 17g

40.   Almond Salad

Ingredients:

½ pear sliced

1 kiwi, peeled and sliced

Few cherry tomatoes, halved

½ cup of wild berries

½ cup of nut mix

½ green bell pepper, sliced

For the dressing:

2 tbsp of honey

¼ cup of fresh lime juice

1 tsp of mustard

Preparation:

Whisk fresh lime juice, mustard and honey with a fork.

In a large bowl, combine the vegetables and add the dressing. Toss well to combine.

If you're not a big fan of fruit/vegetable mixture, you can easily skip the vegetables and create a beautiful fruit salad.

However, you should also replace the mustard dressing with few drops of fresh lemon juice and sugar.

Nutrition information per serving: Kcal: 135, Protein: 1.9g, Carbs: 33.4g, Fats: 0.9g

41.   Mackerel with Potatoes and Greens

Ingredients:

4 medium-sized mackerels, skin on

1 lb of fresh spinach, torn

5 large potatoes, peeled and sliced

¼ cup (divided in half) of extra virgin olive oil

3 garlic cloves, crushed

1 tsp of dried rosemary, finely chopped

2 springs of fresh mint leaves, chopped

1 lemon, juiced

1 tsp of sea salt

Preparation:

Peel and slice potatoes. Make the base layer in a deep, heavy-bottomed pot. Spread one-half of your olive oil over potatoes. Now add torn spinach and top with the remaining olive oil. Add crushed garlic, rosemary, mint, and lemon juice.

Generously sprinkle some salt over mackerels. Make the final layer in your pot and cover.

Cook for 45 minutes over medium-low heat.

Nutrition information per serving: Kcal: 244, Protein: 14g, Carbs: 19.2g, Fats: 12g

42.   Slow Cooked White Beans

Ingredients:

1 lb of white peas

4 slices of dried beef

1 large onion, finely chopped

1 garlic clove, crushed

1 medium-sized red bell pepper, finely chopped

1 small chili pepper, finely chopped

2 tbsp of all-purpose flour

2 tbsp of butter

1 tbsp of cayenne pepper

3 bay leaves, dried

1 tsp of salt

½ tsp of freshly ground black pepper

Preparation:

Melt two tablespoons of butter in a slow cooker. Add chopped onion, crushed garlic, and stir well. Now add dried beef, peas, finely chopped red bell pepper, chili pepper, bay leaves, salt, and pepper. Gently stir in two tablespoons of flour and add three cups of water.

Securely close the lid and cook for 8-9 hours on low setting or 5 hours on high setting.

Nutrition information per serving: Kcal: 210, Protein: 4g, Carbs: 24g, Fats: 12g

43.   Collard Greens Rolls

Ingredients:

1.5 lb of collard greens, steamed

1 lb lean ground beef

2 small onions, peeled and finely chopped

½ cup long grain rice

2 tbsp of olive oil

1 tsp of salt

½ tsp of freshly ground black pepper

1 tsp of mint leaves, finely chopped

Preparation:

Boil a large pot of water and gently the greens. Briefly cook, for 2-3 minutes. Drain and gently squeeze the greens and set aside.

In a large bowl, combine the ground beef with finely chopped onions, rice, salt, pepper, and mint leaves.

Oil a deep pot with some olive oil. Place leaves on your work surface, vein side up. Use one tablespoon of the meat mixture and place it in the bottom center of each leaf. Fold the sides over and roll up tightly. Tuck in the sides and gently transfer to a pot.

Cover and cook for one hour over a medium heat.

Nutrition information per serving: Kcal: 156, Protein: 5.2g, Carbs: 21g, Fats: 7g

44.   Whole Chicken Stew

Ingredients:

1 whole chicken, 3 lbs

10 oz of fresh broccoli

7 oz cauliflower florets

1 large onion, peeled and finely chopped

1 large potato, peeled and chopped

3 medium-sized carrots, sliced

1 large tomato, peeled and chopped

A handful of yellow wax beans, whole

A handful of fresh parsley, finely chopped

¼ cup of extra virgin olive oil

2 tsp of salt

½ tsp of freshly ground black pepper

1 tbsp of cayenne pepper

Preparation:

Clean the chicken and generously sprinkle with some salt. Set aside.

Grease the bottom of a heavy bottomed pot with three tablespoons of olive oil. Add finely chopped onion and stir-fry for 3-4 minutes and then add sliced carrot. Continue to cook for five more minutes.

Now add the remaining oil, vegetables, salt, black pepper, cayenne pepper, and top with chicken. Add one cup of water and cover.

Simmer for one hour over medium heat.

Nutrition information per serving: Kcal: 290, Protein: 31g, Carbs: 39g, Fats: 6g

45. Veal Okra with Artichokes

Ingredients:

7 oz veal shoulder, blade chops

1 lb okra, rinsed and trimmed

3 large artichokes, whole

2 medium-sized tomatoes, halved

2-3 fresh cauliflower florets

2 cups of vegetable broth

A handful of fresh broccoli

3 tablespoons of extra virgin olive oil

1 tsp of Himalayan salt

½ tsp of freshly ground black pepper

Preparation:

Grease a deep pot with three tablespoons of olive oil. Set aside.

Cut each okra pod in half lengthwise and place in a pot. Add tomato halves, artichokes, cauliflower florets, a handful of fresh broccoli, and top with meat chops.

Season with salt and pepper and add two cups of vegetable broth. Give it a good stir and cover.

Cook for 45 minutes over medium-high heat, or two hours over low temperature.

Nutrition information per serving: Kcal: 281, Protein: 19.6g, Carbs: 17.4g, Fats: 15.5g

ADDITIONAL TITLES FROM THIS AUTHOR

70 Effective Meal Recipes to Prevent and Solve Being Overweight: Burn Fat Fast by Using Proper Dieting and Smart Nutrition

By

Joe Correa CSN

48 Acne Solving Meal Recipes: The Fast and Natural Path to Fixing Your Acne Problems in Less Than 10 Days!

By

Joe Correa CSN

41 Alzheimer's Preventing Meal Recipes: Reduce or Eliminate Your Alzheimer's Condition in 30 Days or Less!

By

Joe Correa CSN

70 Effective Breast Cancer Meal Recipes: Prevent and Fight Breast Cancer with Smart Nutrition and Powerful Foods

By

Joe Correa CSN

www.ingramcontent.com/pod-product-compliance
Lightning Source LLC
Chambersburg PA
CBHW051032030426
42336CB00015B/2843